Copyright © 2021

All rights reserved. No part of this book may be reproduced in any form or by any electronic or mechanical means, including information storage and retrieval systems, without permission in writing from the publisher, except by reviewers, who may quote brief passages in a review

Table of Contents

15 Weight Loss Hacks That Actually Work!

Kickstart your weight loss and get healthy with these simple and easy weight loss hacks. These healthy eating hacks will help you to reach your healthy eating goals without feeling deprived of delicious foods……because food is amazing and should be enjoyed!

New beginnings are never easy. They can be scary, full of uncertainty, and overwhelming. But the feeling of doing something that you always wanted to do – whether that's losing weight or living a healthy lifestyle – is definitely worth it.

If you've followed me for any amount of time, you probably already know I'm a firm believer that eating healthy doesn't have to be complicated. I just don't believe you should hate your food just to be "healthy." In my opinion and experience, that will never work because living a tasteless and bland life doesn't sound good to anyone and just can't really be sustainable for the long haul.

In this post, I've shared my best weight loss tips and healthy eating tricks so you'll be able to reach your healthy eating or weight loss goals without giving up tasty foods and snacks. You'll just have to learn some simple healthy food hacks and implement them in your life. It's as simple as it sounds!

EASY NUTRITION HACKS FOR HEALTHY EATING

In an ideal world, we would have time for prepping and cooking balanced meals every day and we would be surrounded by healthy food options. Sadly, we don't live in an ideal world – we live in a busy world and we're surrounded by junk food and other food options that are not nutritious, healthy or good for us. So we need weight loss hacks to keep us on track with our healthy lifestyle. We also need weight loss tips and food hacks for how to get healthy.

But, you know what? You got this! You just have to believe in yourself and try these healthy eating hacks. Trust me, I've made ALL the mistakes. I've also learned, over the course of gaining and losing weight and then eventually keeping it off what works and what doesn't work.

HACK #1: DRINK MORE WATER

Drinking more water will help you to stay hydrated and healthy. Ideally, you'll want to be drinking half your weight, in ounces, every day. For example, I weigh 140 pounds so I should be drinking approximately 70 ounces of water every day — and then more if I exercise. So if you drink around 8 glasses of water a day, that's roughly 60-70 ounces, that's a great goal, and then just adjust for your weight.

Drinking plenty of water isn't only good for hydration — it will help you lose weight, too. Just think about it – water has 0 calories. ZERO. You can drink as much as you want without counting calories.

Water can also help you eat less. Drink a glass of water before a meal. Water will fill up your stomach and you will eat less without feeling hungry. Also — did you know your body tricks you into thinking your hungry when it's actually that you're dehydrated and in need of water? That means, once you drink your water, you'll stop feeling hungry when you're body actually isn't even really hungry.

Finally, drinking water instead of sugary drinks or even sugar-free drinks will also re-train your body and tastebuds to enjoy less sugar each day so you'll crave less sweet treats and empty carbs.

If you need help getting started drinking more water, try to drink a glass of water before any other drink, each time you have a drink during the day. You could also try adding natural flavors to your water, like lemon juice, mint, or fresh fruit slices.

HACK #2: PRACTICE GOOD SLEEP HABITS

Weight loss hacks are not just about food and calories. They are about rest, too. Rest and sleep are just as important for how your body functions and what your body craves. When you sleep well, you have more energy during the day so your body craves less empty carbs and sugar to give you more energy. Have you ever noticed how all you want are sweets and pastries when you're super tired? Yup.

How do you improve your sleeping habits? Here are some quick tips:

• turn off your TV and any electronics at least an hour before going to bed;

• create a sleeping schedule;

• try a relaxing routine (take a bath, read a book, meditate, do yoga) before going to bed to get a good night sleep;

• stop drinking caffeine after 6pm (this one was huge for me);

• start an exercise routine.

The more regular and good sleep your body gets, the happier your body will be, making it easier to get and stay healthy.

HACK #3: COOK YOUR OWN MEALS

A great way to kickstart weight loss and healthy eating is to cook your own food. Cooking your own meals will give you full control over the quality of ingredients, portions, and calories that you put into your body. It's really the first step towards taking control of your food. Eating pre-packed foods are made to keep on shelves, not nourish your body and restaurants liberally use salt and butter to make their food taste great.

This is also a great way for you to learn what healthy foods you like and don't like. If you're looking for healthy eating inspiration, there's TONS of meal prep ideas for healthy eating on this blog to get you started. Food life hacks don't work if you hate your food so find what foods you enjoy and start there with basic ingredient substitutions to make them healthy (more on that later on in this post!).

HACK #4: LEARN TO PORTION CONTROL

Portion sizes are getting larger and larger, despite the need to eat less and less processed foods. Restaurant and takeout portions are way too big. In so many cases, one "portion" can easily exceed your calorie needs for an entire day. And that's why it's important to practice portion control — don't let the restaurant or package dictate your portion size — understand what you need and eat just that.

Now, when I say portion control, I don't mean eating one pea and one carrot for dinner – I mean eat what your body actually needs to function well and stay healthy. The more food you eat that you don't need, the more fat will get stored in your body and vice versa.

So, how do you portion control? Here are some quick tips for how to portion your food:

- eat balanced meals – aim for heavy on the veggies, a few healthy carbs, and lean protein;

- opt for whole grains and complex carbs instead of simple carbs;

- measure food with a kitchen scale to get an understanding of how much you're eating;

- if at a restaurant, take home leftovers (there's no need to clear that giant plate!).

The better you understand what's in your food, the more comfortable you'll become at understanding what your body needs. It might be helpful to track your meals for a typical week to get a baseline for what foods you're eating and how many calories they contain, paying attention to the macros (fat, carb, and protein breakdown). Then, as you understand what foods contain what, you'll be better armed to understand portion control on the fly. Until then, making your food at home is a great way to control the portion.

We also use these meal prep containers to help plan out or meals – if you add the correct amounts to the meal prep container, there's no need to worry about how much of it to eat when you're enjoying your meal.

HACK #5: (MEAL) PLAN AHEAD

In my opinion, planning is the most important weight loss hack out of all weight loss hacks. Without planning, you have very little control over your destiny and healthy lifestyle. There's a saying: "Failing to plan is planning to fail." That means you leave it up to circumstance and fate to find healthy food while out or you deal with what options you have available to you.

Personally, I find it very difficult to eat healthy when I don't have a plan and when I haven't surrounded myself with healthy options. For example, when you have pre-portioned meals ready and waiting for you in the fridge, eating healthy is so much easier. That being said, I do have a post on helpful tips for how to eat healthy at restaurants that you can help to base your decisions on.

Meal planning eliminates temptations almost entirely. Plus, when you meal prep, you can always opt for the best ingredients, you can pre-portion your food and forget about opening the fridge just to find out you have nothing to eat! Check out my post on meal prep ideas to get started.

Planning also helps with making poor food choices. Do you know what restaurant you're going to later? Check out the menu online ahead of time to see what your best options are — it can be difficult to think straight when you're hungry and rushed.

HACK #6: KEEP HEALTHY FOODS CLOSE

It may seem like a no-brainer, but it really helps to keep healthy foods and snacks close by. If you have it near you when you're hungry, you're bound to use it.   That's why unhealthy convenience food is so popular — because people haven't planned. The more foods that are nourishing and healthy for you that you can keep around that's easy to access, the more successful you'll be. This is, of course, assuming you're replacing the unhealthy, pre-packed convenience foods with the healthier options.

Prep grab-and-go bags with minimally processed and low-sugar snacks like…

- nuts;

- dried fruits;

- fresh fruits;

- beef jerky (with low sodium)

- dark chocolate;

- high protein foods, like cottage cheese, hard-boiled eggs, or sustainable canned tuna (packed in water);

• full-fat greek yogurt.

Make grab and go lunch meals such as wraps or mason jar salads and take them at work with you. For busy mornings, prep your breakfast ahead of time just grab it from the fridge or prep freezer smoothie packs and prep your breakfast in 5 minutes in the morning.

HACK #7: USE AN APP

Since we spend a lot of time on our phones and computers, it's probably a good idea to use technology as a healthy food hack, am I right? So look for apps that can help you keep track of your meals, calorie intake, and nutritional profile of your meals. It will be easier to keep track of what you're eating in a day. Or keep a food journal if apps are not your thing.

While I don't recommend calorie-counting as a sustainable part of a healthy lifestyle because it can become tedious and isn't as focused on how your body feels and behaves, apps can be a great way to get a baseline for how much food you're eating and the quality of the food you choose. They can also offer a reference for what foods we eat that make us feel good or bad — and give us a starting point for making positive changes. While there are many options out there, my current fave is MyFitnessPal.

Another great use of using an app is to track how much water you're drinking each day – remember our first hack??

HACK #8: LEARN TO SPOT SUGAR

Identifying the sugar amount and sources in your food is essential to getting healthy. Contrary to what many think , sugar is not just found in desserts, soft drinks, and sweet foods. Sugar is everywhere: in canned food, in junk food, in bread, and even in many snacks that are advertised as healthy. To identify the sugar, make sure you read the label on everything and stay away from anything that has added sugar.

To reduce sugar intake, opt for…

- water instead of sugar-filled drinks;

- homemade sauces instead of canned sauces with lots of sugar;

- whole foods instead of processed foods because processed foods contain added sugar and other ingredients that are not good for you;

- identify the many names of sugar (more on that in this post on how to quit sugar);

- use healthier alternatives for sweeteners, like coconut sugar and raw honey;

- avoid artificial sweeteners

Most of us, after reading the label and seeing high fructose corn syrup as one of the top 5 ingredients in the list would realize that food probably isn't a good choice. But, what if you saw brown sugar, fruit juice, malt syrup, or organic cane juice? Would you stop and think this is just as bad? Because, despite how much nicer they may sound, they're still forms of refined sugar.

Another very easy way to spot sugar in the nutrition labels is by recognizing the "-ose" suffix. So, when you see words that end in -ose, like sucrose, maltose, dextrose, fructose, glucose, galactose, high fructose corn syrup, etc., there's a good chance it is sugar. This is so important, I wrote an entire post on the 7 steps I took to quit sugar which you should check out if you're looking to cut out sugar and get healthy.

HACK #9: SPICE THINGS UP

Nobody wants to eat boring, bland food, especially people wanting to be excited by their healthy lifestyle. Oddly enough, it's very common for people trying to eat healthy to not add spice or flavor to their foods. Personally, I wouldn't last on a diet that didn't taste good, and I would expect anyone else to, either. The whole point of making this healthy change is to change your lifestyle, but if you hate your food, you're never gonna stick with it, in my opinion. I have a full post on how to eat healthy and not hate your food for just this reason.

So, how do you stay clear from unsatisfying, "healthy" foods? Add spice blends, homemade sauces, and marinades to really spice things up and love your healthy lifestyle. That way, you know what's in your food and you get the foods you love, all the while staying healthy and maintaining your goals. Simply put: refuse to suffer through a diet — instead opt for a delicious, healthy lifestyle.

Some of my favorite spices to enhance flavor to get started include:

- sea salt

- ground black pepper

- garlic powder

- onion powder

- cumin

- dried herbs, like rosemary, thyme, oregano, and basil

- cayenne pepper

- cinnamon

- ground ginger

* coconut sugar

Choose the foods you love and find easy replacements for the unhealthy pieces. Find simple swaps to still enjoy your food (more on that with Hack #13!).

HACK #10: SHOP SMART

Okay, so now that you're making your own meals to control the ingredients and portion size, it's also important to buy the right ingredients — mainly to avoid the wrong ones. Fortunately, there are a few simple rules you can follow for a successful and healthy grocery shopping session:

• Follow the perimeter rule – stick to buying groceries from the outer section of the shop and avoiding the inner section. Most fresh and healthy products are situated along the outer perimeter (think produce, dairy, meat and seafood sections), while the packaged, processed foods in the inner perimeter (think sodas, candy, chips, and cookies);

• Make a shopping list – check your pantry and fridge and make a list of healthy ingredients and healthy substitutions for basic ingredients. Make sure to have a plan to follow for what meals you will be making — planning ahead will help you to avoid falling into old habits, like buying teriyaki sauce at the store which is full of sugar and corn syrup instead of making your own homemade teriyaki sauce, for example;

• Try to avoid shopping when you're hungry – you'll buy more ingredients than you need and they won't be healthy! It's very difficult to resist sugary, carby sweets when you're hungry. If you have to, eat a healthy, high-protein snack before heading to the store so your brain is ready to make good choices.

• Shop the sales — this is a great way to save some money while you're shopping so you don't break your bank to get healthy ingredients. Some items, like coconut oil, pure maple syrup, almond butter, and chia seeds can be kinda pricey, so it can help to grab them while they're on sale because you'll be using them often in your cooking.

• Finally, pay special attention to the nutrition labels on everything you buy — yes, this may take some extra time while you're in the store, but it will be very enlightening at just how much sugar, salt, empty/bleached flours, and trans fats get added to the foods you might be used to buying.

In particular, avoid anything with ingredient labels that contain:

• more than 10 ingredients

• added sugar, including: high-fructose corn syrup, corn syrup, evaporated cane juice, cane sugar, aspartame, sugar, and artificial sweeteners

• food coloring, especially Yellow, Blue, Red, and Green

• sodium nitrates and sodium nitrites

- highly processed fats, including: partially hydrogenated oil, palm oil, shortening, and trans fat

- sodium phosphate

- monosodium glutamate (MSG)

- modified food starch

- caramel coloring

- butylated hydroxyanisole (BHA)

In general, you should be able to understand what is in the food and possibly even have the ingredient in your pantry if it's on the label. The farther away from simple, the more to be weary.

HACK #11: USE YOUR BLENDER

If all else fails and you have limited options and limited time to eat healthy, blending your meal can be a great option. From smoothies to protein shakes, you can make any meal filling and nutritious, assuming you're adding healthy ingredients.

For any basic smoothie, all you need is:

• liquid (any unsweetened milk of choice or water)

• fruit (bananas, blueberries, mangos, and strawberries work great)

• fat (can be nut butter, full fat greek yogurt, chia seeds, etc.)

• greens (spinach and kale are easy to blend to get your greens)

• protein powder (can choose to add to make it more filling as a full meal replacement — this protein powder is my fave!)

• ice (only needed if your fruit isn't frozen or to thicken)

If you're looking for a great blender that will never give you problems, definitely check out this Vitamix blender, which is what I have and love.

HACK #12: FORGIVE YOURSELF ALONG THE WAY

Bottom line: you're human, and mistakes happen. If you ever slip up and you indulge in a not-so-healthy meal or snack, forgive yourself! You're are allowed to make mistakes. Living a healthy lifestyle isn't an all-or-noting kinda deal — you'll have great days, but you'll also have not-so-great days. The trick is to just don't let those mistakes take over.

Try to consider this healthy lifestyle as a life-long journey, not a trendy fad. Or as a marathon, not a quick sprint. There will be ups and downs along the way so it's better to stay positive and not blame yourself, but to hold yourself accountable for your choices and always try to improve, within reason.

Making less-than-healthy, unplanned food choices happens to everybody, but it's easy to get back on track if you don't let that mistake turn into a habit or, worse, let that mistake stop you from continuing your otherwise great progress. On a side note, that's what makes planning so valuable — so you don't set yourself up for failure.

HACK #13: FIND HEALTHIER REPLACEMENTS

Important food hacks alert! Fortunately, it is totally possible to enjoy your favorite meals and desserts while you're in the process of losing weight or getting healthy. One of the biggest worries I hear from people not wanting to eat healthier is they are afraid to give up the foods they love so they don't even try. The good news is that you can enjoy almost any food you love by finding a healthier way to make it.

Use healthy alternatives to the ingredients required by your favorite recipes and you'll have no reason to not enjoy those foods. Here are some common healthy alternatives I've used that work great:

• all-purpose flour: whole wheat pastry flour, cassava flour, chickpea flour, almond flour, and coconut flour;

- white sugar or brown sugar: coconut sugar, raw honey, and pure maple syrup;

- butter: coconut oil and olive oil;

- mayo: greek yogurt (for salad dressings) or avocado or hummus for spreading on sandwiches;

- white bread: look for whole wheat sprouted grain bread, like Dave's Killer Bread or Ezekial Bread

- fat-free or reduced-fat foods: choose whole fat foods instead to avoid the processing and increase your fullness

• pasta: there are so many options out there now, including zucchini noodles, veggie noodles, brown rice pasta, quinoa noodles, etc.

HACK #14: CONSIDER INTERMITTENT FASTING

Intermittent fasting can give you a much-needed kick start for weight loss. If you're unfamiliar with fasting, it involves switching between timeframes of eating and now eating (AKA "fasting"). It doesn't mean you don't eat your caloric needs each day, it just means you control the times at which you are eating. This can make it easier to eat larger meals in the middle of the day if you find that you're often hungry all day long.

It takes some time to get used to, especially if you're used to eating 3-4 large meals throughout the day. However, it can be very helpful for getting a handle on your caloric intake so you don't wind up munching all hours of the day. Intermittent fasting isn't for everyone, though, and requires testing to see what works best for you. Typically, one can fast from 6-12 hours of awake time during a day up to even alternating days of time (one day on, one day off).

Intermittent fasting helps with weight loss by:

• Reducing insulin levels, which makes it easier for your body to burn stored fat;

• Increasing human growth hormone (HGH) levels, which help to burn stored fat and grow muscle;

• Lowering blood sugar levels, inflammation, and blood pressure

• Helps to identify goals and follow an easting plan.

Intermittent fasting is not for everyone, and is cautioned against especially for women who are nursing, pregnant, or trying to conceive, people with diabetes or difficulty regulating insulin levels, and people who have eating disorders or medical conditions for which ongoing medication has been prescribed.

So, how does intermittent fasting actually work? Well, personally, I fast from 7pm to 9:30am every day. I make sure to stop consuming anything, except water, after 7pm and I don't eat anything until after my workout, usually around 9:30am. I typically sleep from 11:30pm to 6:30am so I'm fasting while awake for about half the time.

This works really well for me because it allows me to start my day of eating a little later after my workout so I burn up any stored fat even during my workout, which is awesome. I also love how I can eat the same amount of calories as I normally would, but in a more condensed time so it makes me feel more full and less hungry during the day. Then, I resume eating from breakfast, then snack, lunch, and dinner, and start it all over again at 7pm.

HACK #15: INDULGE ON OCCASION!

A very important part of enjoying a healthy lifestyle is balance, not just within each meal with the different macros, but also with how you eat healthy. That's why "cheat meals" or "treat meals" are a welcome option from time to time. No matter how much we love our healthy food, sometimes we crave something that's not healthy. Depriving yourself won't stop your cravings — it might even make them worse. So allow yourself that yummy dessert or the comfort food you crave.

That being said, cheat meals can quickly turn into cheat days, and then it turns into a downward spiral of falling out of whack with your healthy lifestyle. So, here are some tips for how to have a cheat meal without sacrificing your healthy eating goals:

• Pick a timeframe that works for you to go without a cheat meal. For some, that might be one day, and others it might even be one month. Personally, I have a cheat meal each week (every 7 days).

• Save your unhealthy option for that meal, which will help you to look forward to indulging and even over-eating, when it's part of your meal plan.

• Choose a meal that will fill you up and satisfy you — almost to the point of not wanting that meal again for a while. The healthier you eat, the more your healthy body will probably even reject the food you're eating and you may feel gross after eating — this will help to remind you why you have chosen the healthy lifestyle and will shock you right back into shape.

• Stick to just a cheat meal — a cheat day can get out of hand and is too long of a timeframe to go eating unhealthy — it will cause too many bad choices and can easily continue into the next day — the idea is to identify one meal you want, have it, and then move on.

• Allow yourself to enjoy this meal – don't feel bad about it, count the calories, or even think you're cheating on your diet — this is an opportunity for you to loosen the restraints and, in a controlled way, indulge again, which is something those of us on a healthy lifestyle rarely allow ourselves.

- Choose comfort foods, like pizza, pasta, doughnuts, or pancakes and go all out to enjoy the heck out of your meal — you earned it!

Now, you have 15 tried and tested weight loss hacks to help you get and stay healthy. This list is designed to help ease you into a world of eating healthy with as much success as possible. Nothing worth doing is ever too easy, and following a healthy lifestyle is a commitment that takes hard work and dedication, but the results are so worth it.

www.ingramcontent.com/pod-product-compliance
Lightning Source LLC
Chambersburg PA
CBHW052130150726

48002CB00006B/2549